Lupus Recovery without Steroids or Narcotics

The Definitive Beginner's Guide

Table of Contents

Introduction

This book contains proven steps and strategies on how manage and control the symptoms of your lupus disease without resorting to steroids and narcotics. Up to today, medical experts have not yet come up with a known cure for lupus which is a multi-system auto-immune disorder. Traditional medication approaches normally involves the use of corticosteroid, non-steroidal anti-inflammatory drugs or NSAIDs, anti-malarial medications and chemo-therapeutic drugs. Many doctors have questioned the effectiveness of these steroids and narcotics in truly treating the lupus symptoms of patients. More doctors and other health experts have considered using conservative treatment alternatives that do not use steroids and narcotics with positive results. This book aims to provide you with a basic understanding of those alternative treatment methods so you can better decide which option is best for you. But you need to closely work with your doctor in taking medications and other treatments to make sure that your symptoms are properly controlled.

Systemic Lupus Erythematosus is an auto-immune disorder that inflicts a number of complications not only on the person afflicted with the disease but also on his or her family. The causes of lupus are not yet completely known and its manifestations normally vary from one patient to another. To add more complications to the matter, many doctors frequently misdiagnose or overlook the disease.

Doctors make their lupus diagnosis based on the measures disseminated by the American College of Rheumatology or ACR. A patient will only be given a lupus diagnosis when they present at least 4 of the following 11 symptoms:

- Butterfly rashes that normally appear on the cheeks and nose of the patient

- Discold rashes which are thick, disc-like rashes that results to scarring. They normally appear on the body parts that are often exposed to the sun.

- Sensitivity to sunlight which are manifested by rashes after exposure to UVA or UVB light.

- Ulcerations or recurring sores in the mouth are or nose.

- Arthritis which is manifested as swelling of at least 2 peripheral joins coupled with tenderness and generation of fluid.

- Serositis or swelling of the pleura (the lining of the lungs) or of the pericardium (lining of the heart).

- Kidney disorders which are indicated by protein and other abnormal sediments during urine testing.

- Neurologic disorders manifested as a seizure or psychosis that have no other explanations.

- Abnormalities in the blood which are manifested by hemolytic anemia, lowered white blood cell count and lowered platelet count.

- Immune system disorders which are manifested by a positive LE preparation, anti-DNA, and false positive syphilis testing or positive anti-Sm.

- Positive results of ANA blood testing

Thanks again for downloading this book, I hope you enjoy it!

Chapter 1: Overview of Lupus Disease

Lupus can be classified into the following categories:

The symptoms of discoid lupus erythematosus is considered to be cutaneous or restricted to the skin. It is possible for the patient to have either positive or a negative result in an anti-nuclear anti-body (ANA) testing. The symptoms of this type of lupus normally involves mucosal ulcers or inflammations in the nose, mouth and vagina areas, butterfly rashes, rapid losing of hair, thick scars caused by disc shaped lesions, changes in the pigmentation of the skin, hive, welt and Raynaud's phenomena which is characterized by color alterations (from red to white to blue) in the patient's fingertips which is normally a reaction to stress and changes in temperature.

A patient can acquire a drug-induced lupus which is an illness that is distinguished by symptoms that are similar to lupus but actually resulted from bad reactions to certain prescribed medications such carbamazepine which is an anti-convulsion medication. In most cases of drug-induced lupus, the signs and symptoms normally recede when the intake of the specific drugs were discontinued.

When the disorder develops and starts to involve one or several systems in the body, a doctor may already diagnose it as a systemic lupus erythematosus or SLE which can be further broken down into sub-categories depending on the seriousness of the symptoms. The sub-category which does not threaten any organs in the body normally has indications of acute fatigue, dyspnea, high fevers, inflamed gland and joints, muscle pain, joint pain, rashes and other skin ailments. The sub-category which threatens the organs in the body have the same symptoms plus malfunction of one or more organs of the body including the heart, lung, liver and kidney. The prognosis for "organ threatening" SLE is less promising compared to "non-organ threatening" SLE. And the complications of organ threatening SLE normally become terminal.

Even though lupus can occur in all age groups and in all genders, it has been noted that it occurs more often in women who are between 15 and 45 years old. In the U.S. alone, 80 to 92 percent of people suffering from lupus is women. But it has also been noted that drug-induced lupus is not biased on one specific gender because both men and women are evenly susceptible to the disease. There are specific ethnic backgrounds that seem to be more prone to lupus. Those who come from American Indian, African American and Asian ethnicity have the highest incidences of lupus. The Hispanics and the Caucasians come in second place. Geographic location also plays a role in the incidence trends of the disease. It has been reported that there are more people in China and the Philippines who suffer from the disease as compared to Japan.

Chapter 2: Negative Effects of Traditional Lupus Treatments

Lupus presents a major concern to the healthcare experts primarily because there is very inadequate understanding of its causes and progression. The conventional treatment for the disease employs the use of different drug therapies but with inconsistent success. The most common medication prescribed to treat lupus is corticosteroid (e.g. prednisone) with the intention of both suppressing the destructive auto-immune response and stabilizing the ensuing inflammations. Doctors can also prescribe a non-steroidal anti-inflammatory drug (NSAID) to amplify the effects of the corticosteroid medications. Anti-malarial medications (e.g. hydroxychloroquine) may also be prescribed to reduce the symptoms of the disease. Since steroid medications can have negative side effects, some patients are given cyto-toxic drugs (e.g. methotrexate, azathioprine and cyclophosphamide) to reduce the dosage intake of steroid drugs.

Inconsistent outcomes are achieved from these traditional treatment approaches. And patients need to work closely with their doctors to make sure that the side effects do not outweigh the actual symptoms of lupus. Prednisone has been noted to trigger several negative side effects that include complications in the muscular and skeletal systems such as avascular necrosis and Cushinoid symptoms. There have also been a lot of documented cases of gastro-intestinal damage that resulted from excessive intake of NSAID. On the other hand, patients who take cytotoxic medications are not able to attain remission which often leads to side effects including cytopenia, hepatitis A and B, nausea, stomatitis and disturbance in the central nervous system or CNS.

Since traditional medicine still has failed to make any substantial advancement in treating lupus, it is but fitting and reasonable to determine whether alternative treatments and medications can contribute in curing lupus. Currently, the intake of certain vitamins, minerals and fatty acids are considered as valuable in helping treat the symptoms of lupus. Eliminating the foods that trigger or worsen the symptoms from a lupus patient's regular diet was also proven to be an excellent alternative. Additionally, the intake of DHEA and certain Chinese medicines also seem to show healing effects on lupus activities in a patient.

Chapter 3: Lupus Diet and Nutrition

There is actually no specific food that causes lupus and that can treat it. As always, proper nutrition plays a vital role in the overall treatment plan for lupus. Generally, patients suffering from lupus should target a well balanced diet that incorporates a lot of whole grains, fruits and vegetables. Meat, poultry and oily fish can also be included but only in moderate quantities.

If you have been diagnosed with lupus, have a varied and nutritious regular diet can bring the following benefits:

- Reduction in the inflammations caused by the disease and other symptoms

Since lupus is considered an inflammatory disease, it is possible, although it is not yet completely proven, that specific foods that combat inflammation can help in alleviating the symptoms of the disease. On the contrary, the specific foods that trigger inflammation can actually worsen the symptoms of the illness.

The foods that are known to have anti-inflammatory effects are the fruits and vegetables which are enriched with antioxidant substances. Similarly, foods that contain omega 3 fatty acids like oily fish, various nuts, ground flaxseed, canola and olive oils are also believed to combat inflammation.

On the contrary, saturated fats can increase the levels of bad cholesterol in your system that may trigger inflammation. It is therefore ideal to stay away from these foods. Foods that are high in saturated fats include fried dishes, commercially baked food products, creamed soup and sauce, red meats, animal fats, processed meat product, and high fat dairy products (such as whole milk, half and half, cheese, butters and ice cream).

There is one specific food that people with lupus should stay away from and that is alfalfa sprouts. Intake of alfalfa tablets have been reported to have causes flare ups and other lupus-like symptoms such as muscle pains, chronic fatigue, irregular results during blood tests and certain kidney problems. These negative effects are believed to be caused by the body's reaction to a specific amino acid that the alfalfa sprout and seed contain. This specific amino acid can cause the immune system to be activated and thus trigger inflammation in patients suffering from lupus. Some doctors also require their lupus patients to stay away from garlic because it can also cause stimulation of the immune system.

- Maintenance of healthy muscles and strong bones

Whether you have a healthy physical condition or you are suffering from lupus, it is important to have a healthy diet that can help maintain strong bones and muscles. But for patients suffering lupus, this is particularly of a greater concern primarily because the medications prescribed as treatment for the disease can actually heighten your risks of acquiring osteoporosis which is a physical condition wherein the bones in the body have become less dense and can easily be broken.

You need to include foods that are rich in calcium and vitamin D into your regular diet. When you buy dairy items, select those products that have low fat or are fat free such as 1% or half percent skim milks, low fat and low sodium yogurts, and low fat cheese.

But if you are lactose intolerant, you can still have high calcium intake through the following milk options: lactose free, soy and almond. There are also certain juices available in the market which are fortified with calcium and vitamin D.

You can also include a lot of dark green veggies in your diet because they are known to provide high amounts of calcium. But if you are not able to obtain an adequate amount of calcium in your regular diet, you can consult your doctor to ask for a prescription of calcium supplement.

- Resistance against the side effects of medication treatments

The calcium and vitamin D nutrients that we have just discussed can help counterbalance the negative effects of corticosteroid medications which are known to cause damages to the bones. This is just one example of how certain foods can help combat the negative side effects of medication treatments. Another example is a low sodium diet that can help in lessening the body's fluid retention and in lowering blood pressure which are normally both increased when a patient take corticosteroid medicines. Similarly, when your diet includes high amounts of folic acid either from foods such as leafy green vegetables, various fruits and fortified bread and cereal or from folic acid supplements, you can combat the known negative side effects of methotrexate (or Rheumatrex).

When you feel nauseous because of the medications that you take to treat your lupus, it is advisable to have small but frequent meals with foods that are very easy on your digestive system. You can opt to eat dry cereal, bread or crackers. Stay away from foods that are high in grease, spices and acids.

If you also experience upset stomach and irritations when taking corticosteroids and other non-steroidal anti-inflammation medications like ibuprofen or naproxen, you can try taking your medicines with meals to avoid the negative side effects. But always inform your doctors about any discomfort or side effects that you observe when taking medications so he or she can evaluate if there are required changes in your prescription.

- Achievement or maintenance of a healthy weight

As we have discussed in the first chapter, lupus may result to excessive weight gain or loss. It is therefore important that you eat a healthy diet that can help you maintain your healthy or ideal weight.

Rapid weight loss couple with poor appetite are commonly experienced by people who have just received a lupus diagnosis. This may be due to the disease itself or it may be caused by the newly prescribed medication treatments that can give you upset stomach or sores in the mouth. On the other hand, weight gain may result from being inactive after being diagnosed with the disease or from the corticosteroid treatments prescribed to manage the symptoms of the disease.

When you notice that you are experiencing excessive weight loss or weight gain, it is advisable to immediately consult your doctor who can help in assessing your diet and in suggesting a diet program that can help manage your weight. Normally, you will be required to have a low fat diet and regular physical exercise. You can also consult a licensed dietician who can help in designing a customized diet that will fit your specific lifestyle and requirements.

- Reduced risks of heart diseases.

Patients suffering from lupus are known to have higher risks of cardiovascular diseases when compared to other people. It is, therefore, very important that you make sure that your diet is heart-healthy to minimize your risks of acquiring heart problems. You will need to undergo regular tests to help your doctor assess if you have risk factors for cardiovascular diseases that include high blood pressure and high cholesterol. Your doctor may require you to undergo a low fat and low sodium diet and physical exercise to help minimize your risks.

Several research studies also show that omega 3 fatty acids from fish or from fish oils may help in reducing your risks for heart disease. The following foods are good sources of omega 3 fatty acids: salmons, sardines, mackerels, blue fish, herrings, mullets, tuna, halibuts, lake trout, rainbow trout, ground flaxseed, walnut, pecan, healthy oils (canola, walnut and flaxseed).

Chapter 4: Natural Approaches to Lupus Treatment

Alternative treatments for lupus have become more popular than their conventional counterparts because of the inability of the healthcare industry to search for an effective cure for lupus and an increasing patients' desire for a treatment that carries lesser risks of negative side effects.

Dehydroepiandrosterone or DHEA

DHEA is one of the most popular and well-accepted alternative treatment for lupus. It is a steroid molecule that is generated by the cholesterol pregnenolone pathway. It is an intermediary to androstenediol and androstenedione which have potentials to turn to either estrogen or testosterone. The role of DHEA in human physiology is really not yet completely known but there are specific findings that indicate that it can have a helpful part in the pathogenesis of lupus. As we have mentioned in the first chapter, lupus has been noted as a largely female-based illness which is manifested by unusually high amounts of estrogen metabolites and the further lessening of testosterone which naturally have low amounts in females. This indicates that androgens may have an influence in the control of these abnormalities in the hormone levels. Research studies have also shown that the levels of DHEA in the serum of patients with lupus are also low which implies that steroids actually have a deeper link to the illness than what the healthcare experts have predicted. Because of this, medical experts have explored the role of DHEA and its numerous features in numerous research studies.

It was noted that DHEA has several effects in the immune-regulatory system including the enhancement of the production of IL-2 and the ensuing increase in the level of T-helper 1 cells and reduction in the anti-DNA antibody levels in mouse models. When the T-helper 1 cells increase and become dominant, it may result to the lessening of cytokines that trigger inflammations.

A double blind and placebo controlled research study that was performed by van Vollenhoven and company showed that giving DHEA supplements to lupus patients can be beneficial. The DHEA supplement was given at a dosage of 200 mg per day for 3 months to twenty eight females suffering from lupus. The experiment results showed that the level of prednisone was reduced, the incidence of flare ups was lowered and the lupus activity was reduced based on the activity index of SLE disease. The same positive results were not seen with placebo group. In contrary, it was noted that the condition of the patients in the placebo group either remained the same or even deteriorated. The exact reasons why DHEA works is not yet fully comprehended, but it is believed that the positive effect of DHEA is connected to the level of testosterone and the production of IL-2. Medical experts deem that DHEA may have controlled the abnormal levels of these hormones in the patients. It was also noted that patients had good tolerance for the medications with low toxicity levels. But there are still certain side effects that include increased acne and moderate hirsutism that were experienced by some patients. In most cases, the topical steroid medication was considered effective with no patients dropping out of the experiment because of side effects.

Van Vollenhoven and his group conducted another study which aimed to explore the effects of DHEA in a double blind and placebo controlled clinical testing. Lupus patients were chosen in random and were assigned to two different groups for six months - a DHEA group and a placebo group. Both groups were ask to continue with their previous adjunctive medication treatments that mostly included corticosteroid and immuno-suppressives. The exact dosage of the medications given to the patients was not revealed but it confirmed the implication that the differences in dosage are actually negligible. The scientists observed that the patients in the placebo group significantly lost bone density in their lumbosacral spine which was most likely due to the impact of the corticosteroid treatments that they were taking. The patients in the test group were given 200 mg of DHEA per day for 6 months and were noted to have maintained their bone densities for the whole duration of the experiment. This result suggests that DHEA may have an anti-resorptive effect that may counterbalance damages to bones that are caused by corticosteroid medications.

It was also noted that DHEA level is directly correlated to the bone mineral density level in the 150 lupus patient-subjects who were in their pre-menopausal stage. In a research study, it was observed that the subjects who had sufficient serum level of DHEA had notably higher levels of bone mineral density compared to the other subjects who had lower levels of DHEA. The determination of density mass was done by measuring the femoral neck and the lumbar spine. The increase in the patients' bone mineral density indicates that DHEA hormones act as a defence mechanisms that fight early loss of bone density and the ensuing onset osteoporosis. The research study also revealed that the DHEA serum level is inversely related to corticosteroid treatments. The subjects who were given higher dosages of prednisone seemed to have lower levels of DHEA and reduced bone mineral density compared to the patients in the test group. Similar findings were not evident with levels of testosterone, bone mineral density and steroid dose which suggest that DHEA does actually possess these qualities and not any other hormone in the patients' system.

The correlation between DHEA and lupus was further investigated in a one year research study that was conducted on fifty lupus patients that consisted of 37 premenopausal patients and 13 post-menopausal patients who each received 200 mg of DHEA every day and were observed all throughout the course of the research study. Thirty four of the patients were given treatment for 6 months, twenty one of which continued to complete the entire 12 month research study. During the 1st three months of DHEA treatment, the patients started showing enhanced serum levels of DHEA, DHEA sulphate and testosterone. They were able to maintain these increased levels for the rest of the study duration with the continuous intake of the DHEA supplements. But the more important effect of DHEA that was observed during the research study was the reduction in both the prednisone levels and the lupus activity which was measured based on the activity scores of SLE disease. But this is not to say that the research studies only revealed the positive effect of DHEA. It was also observed that 62 percent of premenopausal patients who were part of the research study had more acne as a side effect of the DHEA medication. A few of the patients also acquired mild incidences of hirsutism which is the same observation in van Vollenhoven's research studies. The post-menopausal women also had side effects of acne at a lesser degree but they had more frequency of tenderness in the breasts, alopecia, oiliness in the hair and skin when compared to the women in the pre-menopausal group. The acne which most of the patient-subjects experience were managed by using topical steroid medications.

DHEA Conclusion

The effects of DHEA were also examined to know if it also has an antioxidant property. The medical experts are interested in this particular property because of the great amount of free radicals that damage a lot of the systems and organs within the lupus patient's body. The medical experts believe that extra protection from anti-oxidants will be very valuable for the patients. A research study was performed on lab rats which were either given a diet that lacks vitamin E but has DHEA supplements or a diet that has sufficient amount of vitamin E and still with DHEA supplements. The research study showed that DHEA actually contains anti-oxidants that can decrease the pre-oxidation of iron-induced lipids in the rats that received the vitamin E deficient diet. But the same observations were not noted in the rats that were given a diet with sufficient vitamin E. The medical experts deemed that the anti-oxidant feature of DHEA is existent but they were masked by the vitamin E that was present in the patients' diet. This suggests that the anti-oxidant effects of DHEA may not be apparent if there is sufficient vitamin E in the patient's system. But even if the rats who had vitamin E deficiency may have shown certain anti-oxidant activities, they were also observed to have lost weight and had enlarged kidneys, liver and adrenal glands because of fats. These observations show that DHEA may have the ability to remove free radicals from the body especially if there is an insufficient supply of Vitamin E but it does not seem to exempt vitamin # and stop the indications of deficiency.

Vitamins A and D

Some patients are prescribed to take vitamin A and vitamin E supplements that are fat soluble. One research study was conducted to examine the serum levels of vitamin D in patients with lupus, rheumatoid arthritis and osteoarthritis. It was noted that the vitamin D levels in patients with rheumatoid arthritis and osteoarthritis are in the normal range but was lower in lupus patients. Vitamin D is believed to play an important part in the homeostasis of calcium and in regulating the immune system by inhibiting the activation of lymphocytes and in releasing cytokines. There was no connection found between corticosteroid intake and vitamin D levels which could mean that the low serum level of vitamin D in lupus patients was cause by the disease itself. A likely explanation for the low levels of vitamin D is that since lupus patients have increased sensitivity to sunlight, there is minimal or total lack of exposure to sunlight which results to the low levels of vitamin D. It is therefore important for lupus patients to take vitamin D supplements to fill in the gap.

It has also been observed that giving vitamin supplements at 100,000 IU every day for at least 2 weeks to lupus patients resulted to positive immune system responses in ten women who were participants in a research study that was performed by Dr. Vien. It was also noted that the high dosage of vitamin A did not have any important side effects to the patients and it appeared that the women actually had high tolerances for vitamin A. The noted results of the vitamin A supplements include the enhanced levels of cytotocity which is hormone that is dependent on antibodies and mediated by cells. In addition, it was also noted that the natural killer cell activities were increased as well as the response to IL-2. But the long-term effect of vitamin A supplements and its effect on lupus are not yet completely determined.

Antioxidants

Damages caused by free radicals play an important role in the pathogenesis of lupus. A number of research studies show that antioxidant supplements can improve the condition of lupus patients. It was noted that lupus patients have higher amounts of lipid peroxidase and lower amounts of antioxidants compared to people who have healthier physical conditions. The studies revealed that the following antioxidants - alphatocopherol, beta carotene and retinol - were present in lesser amounts in patients with lupus and rheumatoid arthritis. This revelation suggests that the damages caused by free radicals are a significant factor in the processes of inflammatory disease. This also indicates that patients with lupus and rheumatoid arthritis may need extra antioxidant supplements such as vitamin A, vitamin E and beta carotene.

Traditional Chinese Herbal Medicines

Traditional Chinese doctors have used herbal remedies as the primary medication. One of the most explored herbal plant for the treatment of lupus is Tripterygium wilfordii Hook F or TwHF which is a vine like herbal plant that is grown in the southern region of China. Research studies reveal that TwHF can suppress the production of IL-2, interferon 1 and PGE. But the more apparent positive effects of taking TwHF is the normalization of the symptoms of tiredness, arthralgia, fever and other irregular results of laboratory tests. It was also observed that the prednisone intake of lupus patients can be reduced by at least 50% when they take TwHF.

But you should be aware that even if there are several advantages in taking TwHF, there are certain negative side effects that you should take note of. Patients taking TwHF normally complain of upset stomach, diarrhea, skin rashes and alterations in the pigmentation of their skin. But these negative side effects can actually be managed by adjusting the dosage of the TwHF intake. Most of the symptoms of lupus disappear without much intervention. But there are other negative side effects that are more severe in nature and harder to manage and control such as infertility in male patients that can actually be reversed and amenorrhea in female patients.

There are also some medical experts who are concerned with the toxicity of TwHF especially when there is an overdose. The negative side effects may be related to myocardial, intestinal damages and renal failure. In order for you to fully take advantage of the benefits of TwHF, it is important that you closely monitor your dosage intake to prevent any toxic results.

Other popular Chinese herbal remedies include Atractylodes ovata, Angelica sinensis, Cordyceps sinensis, Ligustrum lucidum and Coodonopsis pilosula.

Conclusion

Thank you again for downloading this book!

I hope this book was able to help you to learn the different treatment options that you have to cure your lupus.

The next step is to consult your doctor and discuss which alternatives are best for you.

Finally, if you enjoyed this book, please take the time to share your thoughts and post a review on Amazon. It'd be greatly appreciated!

Thank you and good luck!

www.ingramcontent.com/pod-product-compliance
Lightning Source LLC
Chambersburg PA
CBHW051830170526
45167CB00005B/2221